My Sacred Heart Diet
How I lost 42 Pounds in 2 weeks!

By Victor Bahamonde

authorHOUSE®

AuthorHouse™
1663 Liberty Drive, Suite 200
Bloomington, IN 47403
www.authorhouse.com
Phone: 1-800-839-8640

First published by AuthorHouse 5/22/2009

ISBN: 978-1-4389-8948-8 (e)
ISBN: 978-1-4389-8745-3 (sc)
ISBN: 978-1-4389-8746-0 (hc)

Printed in the United States of America
Bloomington, Indiana

This book is printed on acid-free paper.

About The Book

In this book, Victor Bahamonde shares his story of how he lost 42 pounds in just 14 days and 61 pounds in 28 days.

Over this time he has learned new and simple techniques on eating naturally healthy foods resulting in maximum weight loss in a short amount of time. His weight loss program details specifically everything needed for success in losing weight naturally, quickly and permanently.

He points out how mistakes are made by people in their every day lives resulting in excessive weight gain unnecessarily. His concepts are easy to understand and implement.

DEDICATION

I thank all of my children, family and friends for all their positive support and encouragement I was given during this weight loss journey. With all your positive motivation I was inspired to lose all the excessive weight and write this book to help others like me.

I also thank my Mom and Dad for their unconditional love and support.

I dedicate this book to my beloved lifetime partner Ivonne, who has made my life wonderful, beautiful and meaningful. *"Behind every great man there is a great woman."*

Here Is My Story

My name is Victor Bahamonde. I am forty four years old and originally from Crown Heights in Brooklyn, New York. I was a New York City Corrections Officer for eleven years at Rikers Island Correctional Complex. I moved to Orlando Florida in the summer of 2000 to get away from the cold weather. I still miss New York City especially since I have a lot of family still living there. Orlando Florida on the other hand is a great place to raise a family. Especially with the blue skies, green landscape, amusement parks and the beautiful lakes and beaches close by. I am married to my wonderful wife of twenty eight years with four beautiful children. My Sons are seven and twenty one years old. My Daughters are fifteen and twenty six years old. I also have a grandson who is three years old.

I have always been very healthy no matter what I have eaten in the past. I love rice, meat, seafood, bread, potatoes, fried food, fruits, vegetables and junk food. Orange juice was my water. I rarely drank water. You name it, I love it. Italian, Japanese, Chinese, Spanish, Mediterranean, French and of course American fast food. All you can eat buffets, even better.

Suddenly in February of 2009 I went to the doctor for a cold. My blood pressure for the first time in my life was 145 over 120. I was experiencing nasty headaches that I never had before. I ignored it thinking it was due to the cold I had. About a week later I was at the supermarket. They had a blood pressure machine by the pharmacy so that anyone can check their blood pressure for free. I checked mine and again it was high at 141 over 118. I couldn't believe that I was now a high blood pressure patient.

I was very mad at myself going from 175 pounds to 283 pounds in 20 years. I slowly but surely got heavier every year. I then knew that my weight was beginning to make me sick and diseased. I never had any health issues until now. I was also getting severe headaches which I learned was due to the high blood pressure. I am not an advocate for fixing health problems with pills unless you can't do anything about it.

In early March 2009 my wife said to me, "Let's go on this diet I heard about". I agreed, but when I read it, I found it to be boring, unspecific and distasteful. I started my own weight loss program and as of day 14, I have lost 42 pounds in which I now weigh 241 pounds from my original 283 pounds. Now as of day 28 I have lost a total of 61 pounds. I now weigh 222 pounds from my original weight of 283 pounds.

I was really determined to lose the weight or pay the price with a heart attack, high blood pressure, diabetes, etc. I refused to take any high blood pressure medication that can cause all types of side effects including sexual deficiencies to say the least. I am strong, healthy, and still very much interested in sex. I wasn't going to let laziness, ignorance or lack of will power to conquer me. My life depended on losing the weight and having a more natural, healthy life style.

That is exactly what this weight loss program is, a healthy life style change. I realized that not only I was under active and not exercising regularly. I was also eating too much processed foods, soda and junk food. I was over eating constantly at all types of fancy restaurants, fast food restaurants and at home.

If it was served, it was all consumed. At home my motto was, "seconds or thirds please." I had that same motto at all the cruise and all inclusive resort vacations I went to also.

My oldest Son would always ask me, "Dad, why are you breathing and sweating heavily every time I help you." "You never use to breathe and sweat profusely like this before." I would be terribly embarrassed and say nothing. I knew my excessive weight was causing me severe fatigue even when accomplishing minimal tasks. Now that I have lost a lot of the weight. All of the fatigue, heavy breathing and sweating I use to experience during minimal and normal tasks are completely gone!

Due to this healthy eating and exercising life style change. I have not only lost a lot of weight and toned down my body. But most of all, my headaches are gone and my blood pressure is at 108 over 75. That is what it used to be always.

I am also very happy about fitting into my clothes that where too tight on my waist. I was a 47 waist squeezing into a size 42 and 44 waist clothes. Now I am a 40 waist. I use to wear 3X size clothes, now I wear L size clothes. Keep in mind I am 6 foot 1 inches tall. I also had to drape my shirts outside of my pants to camouflage my "beer belly". For the record I rarely drank beer. Now I tuck all my shirts into my pants which I can see for myself that I look great.

It feels great to know that I look and feel "normal". It is amazing how I took for granted good health and how I perceived being extremely over weight as a variation of normal. Especially since there are so many people in the world that are extremely over weight. I believed I wasn't one of "those" overweight people. In reality I was definitely over weight and in denial. Now I'm not in denial anymore and also not overweight anymore.

All I wanted to accomplish is that I look great and feel great, so that I can be great at whatever I desire to be or do. And not let negativity surround me. Life is too short to be sick, unhealthy, overweight and lazy unless I can't do anything about. If I can do something about it, I will.

My life, my wife, my children, my grandchildren depend on me. I will not shorten my life span due to something I could have changed in the normal course of my day.

I see my life in a very, very positive way. I am filled with joy and happiness knowing I have self improved myself for my benefit first. My family's benefit second. My business benefit third. My wife recently complemented me by stating, "Wow, you look so young." And my oldest daughter also complemented me by stating, "Dad, you now look like when I was a little girl, it is like seeing you back in time." Remember my oldest daughter is 26 years old. And she gave me a compliment I wasn't prepared for. I then looked at myself closely in the mirror and I have to strongly agree that I not only feel younger, but I look a lot younger!

Do not shorten your life span due to something you could have changed in the normal course of your day!

As with anything you do in life. Do it with a sense of urgency! Don't do it just to do it. Complete the tasks deliberately, intentionally and as perfect as you can achieve it. All while having fun knowing you are burning calories and losing weight deliberately and intentionally.

Look great, feel great, and be great!

Learn to love and respect your body for what it is, a gift from God. Take care of this God given gift.

Because no one but <u>you</u> can take care of it better!

My Sacred Heart Diet

This 7 day weight loss program can be used continuously and as often as you like. If correctly followed, it will flush out your digestive system of impurities and give you a feeling of well being. After only 7 days on this weight loss program, you will begin to be lighter by at least 10 to 17 pounds, feel less bloated and experience an abundance of energy. With a little motivation you can achieve a new healthy lifestyle while reaping the rewards of good health and the natural process of weight loss attributed to it.

The Soup

Soup ingredients:

2 large tomatoes
3 large green onions (chives)
1 large 64 ounce can or carton of beef or chicken broth (no fat)
1 bunch of celery
2 pounds of green beans
2 pounds of carrots
2 green peppers
16 ounces of water

If you can afford it, try to buy everything organic. I am a great believer in organic food. The least processing of our food intake. The better our digestive system will appreciate it. Our bodies weren't made to consume additives, steroids, antibiotics, pesticides or preservatives.

But if you are on a very tight budget, canned or non organic food is ok also. On the other hand. Since you'll be saving money on groceries and restaurants, why not invest the savings into organic food. Just food for thought.

Cut the vegetables into small to medium pieces. Then add the vegetables and 1 large 64 ounce can or carton of beef or chicken broth (no fat) with 16 ounces of water into a soup pot and bring to a fast boil for 10 minutes. Then reduce to a simmer and continue to cook until all the vegetables are tender. Season the soup as desired with salt, pepper, curry, parsley, fresh cilantro (finely chopped), hot sauce or Worcestershire sauce to your taste.

This soup can be eaten anytime you are hungry during the week. Eat as much as you want, whenever you want. This soup is nutritious and very low in calories. Fill a thermo or a microwavable container in the morning and take it with you. Especially, if you plan on being away from home during the day or going to work or school.

In a couple of days the soup will also help you in curving your appetite. A lot of discipline and determination is involved with staying on track with this weight loss program.

DO NOT EAT

No bread, alcohol, carbonated drinks, (including zero or low calorie diet drinks). A rule of thumb is eating nothing that is white in color except for cauliflower. Remember, absolutely no fried foods or any alcoholic beverages.

Unless your religion requires it, I suggest you keep the wine consumption down to a minimum at 4 ounces or less per day until you have reached your desired weight.

EAT & DRINK EVERY DAY

Drink 4 to 8 glasses of water per day, as well in addition to any combination of the following:

Hot soup as much as you desire

Black coffee (no sugar or sugar substitutes)

Tea (no sugar or sugar substitutes)

Unsweetened fruit juices

Unsweetened cranberry juice (surprisingly it's very naturally sweet and you can mix it with water and ice)

Skim milk (Lactaid fat free milk, if you are lactose intolerant)

Bran cereal, preferably Fiber One brand (surprisingly, it really tastes good).

DAY ONE

Eat only hot soup and fruit today.

Eat any fruit (except bananas) today. Cantaloupes and watermelon are lower in calories than most other fruits. You can even make a fruit smoothie with ice or Skim milk (Lactaid fat free milk, if you are lactose intolerant).

Eat slowly, thoroughly taste and enjoy your food. Take small bites or slice the fruit in order to give time for your brain to tell you that you are full.

Eat the soup as hot as possible. This will also make you eat it slowly giving your brain time to tell you are full.

DAY TWO

Eat any vegetables, they can be raw, cooked, canned or steamed. Eat a green leafy vegetable salad with sliced cucumbers, sliced tomatoes and a dash of salt. Stay away from dry beans, peas or corn. Eat the vegetables with the hot soup or add the vegetables to the hot soup to make it heartier. You can even have freshly blended vegetable juice.

Eat the soup as hot as possible. This will also make you eat it slowly giving your brain time to tell you are full.

At dinner time enjoy a big baked potato with butter. Do not eat any fruits today.

Eat slowly, thoroughly taste and enjoy your food.

DAY THREE

Eat all the soup, fruit, and vegetables you want today. You can have a leafy green vegetable salad with sliced cucumbers, sliced tomatoes, dried cranberries and dressed with a fresh squeezed lemon or orange juice. You can even have a fruit smoothie with ice or Skim milk (Lactaid fat free milk, if you are lactose intolerant) or freshly blended vegetable juice. No baked potato.

Eat slowly, thoroughly taste and enjoy your food. Take small bites of the fruit or slice in order to give time for your brain to tell you that you are full.

Eat the soup as hot as possible. This will also make you eat it slowly giving your brain time to tell you are full.

If you have followed the program without cheating, you will have realized that you should have lost 5-7 pounds.

This is just the beginning of your weight loss journey. Stay on track for four more days and amaze your friends, family and coworkers. But most of all, amaze yourself!

DAY FOUR

Eat at least 3 bananas with as much skim milk (Lactaid fat free milk, if you are lactose intolerant) you desire. With a cup of bran or fiber if desired in a bowl for breakfast. Eat plenty of the hot soup. You can even have a banana smoothie with ice or Skim milk (Lactaid fat free milk, if you are lactose intolerant).

Eat slowly, thoroughly taste and enjoy your food. Take small bites of the banana or slice in order to give time for your brain to tell you that you are full.

Eat soup as hot as possible. This will also make you eat it slowly giving your brain time to tell you are full.

DAY FIVE

Eat 10 to 20 ounces of beef, fish or chicken (no skin) with as many as 6 tomatoes today. You can even have freshly blended tomato juice or a sliced tomato salad with a dash of salt. Eat the hot soup at least once today.

Eat slowly, thoroughly taste and enjoy your food. Take small bites of the beef, fish or chicken (no skin) in order to give time for your brain to tell you that you are full.

Eat the soup as hot as possible. This will also make you eat it slowly giving your brain time to tell you are full.

DAY SIX

Eat all the beef, fish or chicken (no skin) with vegetables to your hearts content. You can even have 2-3 lean steaks (trim the fat off) with a green leafy vegetable salad with sliced cucumbers, sliced tomatoes and a dash of salt. No baked potato. Eat the hot soup at least once today.

Eat slowly, thoroughly taste and enjoy your food. Take small bites of the beef, fish or chicken (no skin) in order to give time for your brain to tell you that you are full.

Eat the soup as hot as possible. This will also make you eat it slowly giving your brain time to tell you are full.

DAY SEVEN

Eat all the brown rice and raw, cooked, canned or steamed vegetables with a glass of unsweetened fruit juice. You can even eat brown rice vegetable sushi with a dash of soy sauce. Or you can have freshly blended vegetable juice or a green leafy salad with sliced cucumbers, sliced tomatoes and a dash of salt. Eat the hot soup at least once today.

Eat slowly, thoroughly taste and enjoy your food.

Eat the hot soup as hot as possible. This will make you eat it slowly giving your brain time to tell you are full.

By the end of the 7ᵗʰ day if you have not cheated on the weight loss program. You should have lost 10 to 17 pounds.

If you lost more than 17 pounds, stay off the weight loss program for 1 day before resuming the program again. Use the "eat slow and small principle" to prevent over eating.

Continue the weight loss program as long as it takes for you to achieve your desired weight. You will feel an abundance of energy. Mentally you will be very sharp.

Physically your knees, hips and back will feel better due to the weight loss lessening the pressure and stress on those joints.

Cheating & Binging Triggers

Cheating

If for any reason you are anticipating cheating or just happen to cheat by accident. Use the, "eat slow and small" principle in order to prevent you from over eating. Try not to cheat for more than two days consecutively in order to prevent a major disruption in this weight loss diet. Don't worry, be happy. Tomorrow is another day when you can start where you left off. Failure is when you have completely given up. So don't give up, and continue where you left off. Just because other people choose to eat unhealthy doesn't mean you should eat unhealthy. Remember this is a healthy life style change. It will take time and discipline to achieve your desired weight. The more discipline, the greater the reward.

Binging Triggers

Another important aspect to achieving your weight loss to a desired weight that fits best with your body type is keeping away from what I call, "binging triggers". Stress, negative people and being antisocial are all "binging triggers" that can give you incentive to cheat or quit your weight loss program. Stay away from negative people, don't be antisocial, and avoid stress when possible. We all have a natural tendency to run to food when we are not happy. This is very, very counter productive. If you need relief, eat something that you have to consume slow, under the "eat small and slow" principle. Like the very hot soup, raw vegetables, freshly blended fruit smoothie with ice or Skim milk (Lactaid fat free milk, if you are lactose intolerant), freshly blended vegetable juice, a green leafy salad or sliced fruit.

Do not consume processed foods, soda, alcoholic beverages or junk food. Experience the episode by restructuring your eating habits in order to maintain your healthy life style.

Be strong! But most of all, be STRONG and SMART. With the two combined you can weather the episode in a positive manner TO YOUR ADVANTAGE.

Increasing Daily Activity & Exercise

Include aerobic exercise in your normal activities during the course of the day or night. This will keep you trim since you will be losing weight pretty fast. Twenty minutes per day of aerobic exercise is more than enough. Too much exercise will make your body build muscle at your current weight and keep you there. So don't over exercise. These 20 minutes of exercise per day will increase your metabolism resulting in burning more calories and losing more weight. Push ups, sit ups, pull ups, squats, treadmill or punching bag (if you have one) and aerobic videos are just as good. Play tennis, basketball, volleyball, hockey, football, bicycling, baseball or just catch is a great exercise. The gym is not necessary. So save your time and money if you desire. Remember to stretch first for 5 minutes.

I have noticed that the number one reason we all gain weight is due to the fact that we are not as active as we use to be.

Walk more, during lunch (bring your walking sneakers to work), to and from work, to church, to the supermarket (only if you are buying light groceries), at the park, at the zoo, at the beach or the lake (swimming is also great exercise if you know how to), or take your dog for a long walk.

Ride your bicycle to the supermarket, church, work, to run errands, to the doctors or dentist office or just for a spin around your neighborhood.

Swimming in the pool, lake and ocean is great exercise if you know how to swim. Snorkeling and scuba diving is also very fun if you know how to swim. These are all great exercises especially since you use all the muscles in your body with very little impact on your knees and back.

Go to parties (engagement, weddings, birthdays, sweet sixteen, wedding anniversaries, Thanksgiving, Christmas, New Years Eve) or dance clubs and become more social with no consumption of alcoholic beverages. That is where you will find a great exercise that everyone should do as much as possible. Dancing of course. Drink plenty of water if you desire it. This exercise is fun and you will give your body a total workout. Remember, the more you dance, the better you will be at it. Have your meal and soup prior to going to reduce any temptation if necessary.

Then there is other calorie burning activities at home like spring cleaning, painting the outside of the house, painting the inside of the house, vacuuming all the carpets and mopping the floors, steam cleaning all the carpets, washing the windows, power washing the pool deck or patio, washing and grooming the cat or dog, practicing dancing in your living room by yourself or with your partner, rearranging your furniture, landscaping your property, cleaning your car inside and out, cleaning out the garage or storage closet, completing your TO DO list.

As with anything you do in life. Do it with a sense of urgency! Don't do it just to do it. Complete the tasks deliberately, intentionally and as perfect as you can achieve it. All while having fun knowing you are burning calories and losing weight deliberately and intentionally.

Dining at Restaurants

If you are going out to eat with family or friends. I have a simple over eating cutting principle. When you order your entrée at the restaurant ask the waiter to split the serving of one person for two separately before they serve the food. That way you can share with a friend or family member. Another option would be to have the split portion of the entrée to go so that you can take it home and eat it in another day. This avoids having the whole portion of the entrée served to you. Reducing the temptation of eating the whole portion, instead now you can enjoy half the portion. Restaurants typically have large portions with high calories. This principle cuts the fat, carbohydrates and calories in half with ease while letting you eat all the food on your plate stress free.

Stay away from all alcoholic beverages. Alcoholic beverages inhibit your diet discipline and will likely lead to unhealthy eating and over eating. In other words, we tend to lose control of our diet when alcohol is consumed. That is in addition to the high calories the alcoholic beverages have. A simple glass of water with a lemon wedge is a great way to keep on track while dining out.

As far as desserts are concerned. Stay away from all of the desserts unless it is a fresh fruit salad. Deserts typically are very high in calories, fat and sugar. Desserts are to be avoided as a rule of thumb.

Maintaining Your New Weight

When you have finally achieved your desired weight for your body type. Continue to eat all natural and healthy foods (preferably organic in order to stay away from additives, steroids, antibiotics, pesticides or preservatives.) and exercise daily for at least 20 minutes or more per day. Both of these tips are very important in order to maintain your new weight. If you do consume processed, artificially made or fried foods continually, start this weight loss program again the following day in order to flush out all the impurities from your body.

Your body may flush itself out automatically any way. Why? Because you have cleaned out your digestive system and replaced it with all natural foods that it was designed to digest. When something fried, processed or artificially made is consumed. Your body knows it and starts to flush all the impurities out of your body automatically, only if you have completed this weight loss program for at least 7 days. If you must cheat, do it wisely not foolishly. In other words be very selective in what you are eating in order to minimize the calories, fat and sugar consumed. Then just simply start the weight loss program again the following day where you left off until you are back to your desired weight.

I bid you all success on your journey to a great healthy life style change which results in improved health and your desired weight loss.

Do not shorten your life span due to something you could have changed in the normal course of your day!

As with anything you do in life. Do it with a sense of urgency! Don't do it just to do it. Complete the tasks deliberately, intentionally and as perfect as you can achieve it. All while having fun knowing you are burning calories and losing weight deliberately and intentionally.

Look great, feel great, and be great!

Learn to love and respect your body for what it is, a gift from God. Take care of this God given gift.

BECAUSE NO ONE BUT <u>YOU</u> CAN TAKE
CARE OF IT BETTER!

I HAVE ENCLOSED IN THE FOLLOWING PAGES A MINIATURE VERSION OF THE DIET SO YOU CAN PUT IT ON YOUR REFRIGERATOR FOR QUICK REFERENCING.

The Soup

Soup ingredients:

2 large tomatoes
3 large green onions (chives)
1 large 64 ounce can or carton of beef or chicken broth (no fat)
1 bunch of celery
2 pounds of green beans
2 pounds of carrots
2 green peppers
16 ounces of water

If you can afford it, try to buy everything organic. I am a great believer in organic food. The least processing of our food intake. The better our digestive system will appreciate it. Our bodies weren't made to consume additives, steroids, antibiotics, pesticides or preservatives.

But if you are on a very tight budget, canned or non organic food is ok also. On the other hand. Since you'll be saving money on groceries and restaurants, why not invest the savings into organic food. Just food for thought.

Cut vegetables into small to medium pieces. Then add the vegetables and 1 large 64 ounce can or carton of beef or chicken broth (no fat) with 16 ounces of water into a soup pot and bring to a fast boil for 10 minutes. Then reduce to a simmer and continue to cook until vegetables are tender. Season with salt, pepper curry, parsley, fresh cilantro (finely chopped), hot sauce or Worcestershire sauce if desired to your taste.

This soup can be eaten anytime you are hungry during the week. Eat as much as you want, whenever you want. This soup is nutritious and very low in calories. Fill a thermo or a microwavable container in the morning and take it with you. Especially, if you plan on being away from home during the day or going to work or school.

In a couple of days the soup will also help you in curving your appetite. A lot of discipline and determination is involved with staying on track with this weight loss program.

<u>DO NOT EAT</u>

-

No bread, alcohol, carbonated drinks, (including zero or low calorie diet drinks). A rule of thumb is eating nothing that is white in color except for cauliflower. Remember, absolutely no fried foods or any alcoholic beverages.

Unless your religion requires it, I suggest you keep the wine consumption down to a minimum at about 4 ounces or less per day until you have reached your desired weight.

EAT & DRINK EVERY DAY

Drink 4 to 8 glasses of water per day, as well in addition to any combination of the following:

Hot soup as much as you desire

Black coffee (no sugar or sugar substitutes)

Tea (no sugar or sugar substitutes)

Unsweetened fruit juices

Unsweetened cranberry juice (surprisingly it's very naturally sweet and you can mix it with water and ice)

Skim milk (Lactaid fat free milk, if you are lactose intolerant)

Bran cereal, preferably Fiber One brand (surprisingly, it really tastes good).

DAY ONE

Eat only hot soup and fruit today.

Eat any fruit (except bananas) today. Cantaloupes and watermelon are lower in calories than most other fruits. You can even make a fruit smoothie with ice or Skim milk (Lactaid fat free milk, if you are lactose intolerant).

Eat slowly, thoroughly taste and enjoy your food. Take small bites or slice the fruit in order to give time for your brain to tell you that you are full.

Eat the soup as hot as possible. This will also make you eat it slowly giving your brain time to tell you are full.

DAY TWO

Eat any vegetables, they can be raw, cooked, canned or steamed. Eat a green leafy vegetable salad with sliced cucumbers, sliced tomatoes and a dash of salt. Stay away from dry beans, peas or corn. Eat the vegetables with the hot soup or add the vegetables to the hot soup to make it heartier. You can even have freshly blended vegetable juice.

Eat the soup as hot as possible. This will also make you eat it slowly giving your brain time to tell you are full.

At dinner time enjoy a big baked potato with butter. Do not eat any fruits today.

Eat slowly, thoroughly taste and enjoy your food.

DAY THREE

Eat all the soup, fruit, and vegetables you want today. You can have a leafy green vegetable salad with sliced cucumbers, sliced tomatoes, dried cranberries and dressed with a fresh squeezed lemon or orange juice. You can even have a fruit smoothie with ice or Skim milk (Lactaid fat free milk, if you are lactose intolerant) or freshly blended vegetable juice. No baked potato.

Eat slowly, thoroughly taste and enjoy your food. Take small bites of the fruit or slice in order to give time for your brain to tell you that you are full.

Eat the soup as hot as possible. This will also make you eat it slowly giving your brain time to tell you are full.

If you have followed the program without cheating, you will have realized that you should have lost 5-7 pounds.

This is just the beginning of your weight loss journey. Stay on track for four more days and amaze your friends, family and coworkers. But most of all, amaze yourself!

DAY FOUR

Eat at least 3 bananas with as much skim milk (Lactaid fat free milk, if you are lactose intolerant) you desire. With a cup of bran or fiber if desired in a bowl for breakfast. Eat plenty of the hot soup. You can even have a banana smoothie with ice or Skim milk (Lactaid fat free milk, if you are lactose intolerant).

Eat slowly, thoroughly taste and enjoy your food. Take small bites of the banana or slice in order to give time for your brain to tell you that you are full.

Eat soup as hot as possible. This will also make you eat it slowly giving your brain time to tell you are full.

DAY FIVE

Eat 10 to 20 ounces of beef, fish or chicken (no skin) with as many as 6 tomatoes today. You can even have freshly blended tomato juice or a sliced tomato salad with a dash of salt. Eat the hot soup at least once today.

Eat slowly, thoroughly taste and enjoy your food. Take small bites of the beef, fish or chicken (no skin) in order to give time for your brain to tell you that you are full.

Eat the soup as hot as possible. This will also make you eat it slowly giving your brain time to tell you are full.

DAY SIX

Eat all the beef, fish or chicken (no skin) with vegetables to your hearts content. You can even have 2-3 lean steaks (trim the fat off) with a green leafy vegetable salad with sliced cucumbers, sliced tomatoes and a dash of salt. No baked potato. Eat the hot soup at least once today.

Eat slowly, thoroughly taste and enjoy your food. Take small bites of the beef, fish or chicken (no skin) in order to give time for your brain to tell you that you are full.

Eat the soup as hot as possible. This will also make you eat it slowly giving your brain time to tell you are full.

DAY SEVEN

Eat all the brown rice and raw, cooked, canned or steamed vegetables with a glass of unsweetened fruit juice. You can even eat brown rice vegetable sushi with a dash of soy sauce. Or you can have freshly blended vegetable juice or a green leafy salad with sliced cucumbers, sliced tomatoes and a dash of salt. Eat the hot soup at least once today.

Eat slowly, thoroughly taste and enjoy your food.

Eat the hot soup as hot as possible. This will make you eat it slowly giving your brain time to tell you are full.

By the end of the 7th day if you have not cheated on the weight loss program. You should have lost 10 to 17 pounds.

If you lost more than 17 pounds, stay off the weight loss program for 1 day before resuming the program again. Use the "eat slow and small principle" to prevent over eating.

Continue the weight loss program as long as it takes for you to achieve your desired weight. You will feel an abundance of energy. Mentally you will be very sharp.

Physically your knees, hips and back will feel better due to the weight loss lessening the pressure and stress on those joints.

Use the following pages to document your progression to your desired weight.

Document everything you eat and all your calorie burning activities and exercise.

This is very important in order to keep you honest to yourself and keep you on track of your goal.

Daily Journal Of Your Weight Loss Progress

Day One

Daily Journal Of Your Weight Loss Progress

Day Two

DAILY JOURNAL OF YOUR WEIGHT LOSS PROGRESS

DAY THREE

Daily Journal Of Your Weight Loss Progress

Day Four

Daily Journal Of Your Weight Loss Progress

Day Five

Daily Journal Of Your Weight Loss Progress

Day Six

Daily Journal Of Your Weight Loss Progress

Day Seven

Daily Journal Of Your Weight Loss Progress

Day Eight

Daily Journal Of Your Weight Loss Progress

Day Nine

Daily Journal Of Your Weight Loss Progress

Day Ten

Daily Journal Of Your Weight Loss Progress

Day Eleven

Daily Journal Of Your Weight Loss Progress

Day Twelve

Daily Journal Of Your Weight Loss Progress

Day Thirteen

Daily Journal Of Your Weight Loss Progress

Day Fourteen

Daily Journal Of Your Weight Loss Progress

Day Fifteen

Daily Journal Of Your Weight Loss Progress

Day Sixteen

Daily Journal Of Your Weight Loss Progress

Day Seventeen

Daily Journal Of Your Weight Loss Progress

Day Eighteen

Daily Journal Of Your Weight Loss Progress

Day Nineteen

Daily Journal Of Your Weight Loss Progress

Day Twenty

DAILY JOURNAL OF YOUR WEIGHT LOSS PROGRESS

DAY TWENTY ONE

Daily Journal Of Your Weight Loss Progress

Day Twenty Two

Daily Journal Of Your Weight Loss Progress

Day Twenty Three

Daily Journal Of Your Weight Loss Progress

Day Twenty Four

Daily Journal Of Your Weight Loss Progress

Day Twenty Five

Daily Journal Of Your Weight Loss Progress

Day Twenty Six

Daily Journal Of Your Weight Loss Progress

Day Twenty Seven

Daily Journal Of Your Weight Loss Progress

Day Twenty Eight

DAILY JOURNAL OF YOUR WEIGHT LOSS PROGRESS

DAY TWENTY NINE

Daily Journal Of Your Weight Loss Progress

Day Thirty

Daily Journal Of Your Weight Loss Progress

Day Thirty One

Daily Journal Of Your Weight Loss Progress

Day Thirty Two

Daily Journal Of Your Weight Loss Progress

Day Thirty Three

Daily Journal Of Your Weight Loss Progress

Day Thirty Four

Daily Journal Of Your Weight Loss Progress

Day Thirty Five

DAY THIRTY SIX

Daily Journal Of Your Weight Loss Progress

Day Thirty Seven

DAY THIRTY EIGHT

Daily Journal Of Your Weight Loss Progress

Day Thirty Nine

Daily Journal Of Your Weight Loss Progress

Day Forty

Daily Journal Of Your Weight Loss Progress

Day Forty One

Daily Journal Of Your Weight Loss Progress

Day Forty Two

Daily Journal Of Your Weight Loss Progress

Day Forty Three

Daily Journal Of Your Weight Loss Progress

Day Forty Four

Daily Journal Of Your Weight Loss Progress

Day Forty Five

DAY FORTY SIX

Daily Journal Of Your Weight Loss Progress

Day Forty Seven

Daily Journal Of Your Weight Loss Progress

Day Forty Eight

DAY FORTY NINE

DAY FIFTY

Daily Journal Of Your Weight Loss Progress

Day Fifty One

Daily Journal Of Your Weight Loss Progress

Day Fifty Two

Daily Journal Of Your Weight Loss Progress

Day Fifty Three

Day Fifty Four

Daily Journal Of Your Weight Loss Progress

Day Fifty Five

Daily Journal Of Your Weight Loss Progress

Day Fifty Six

Daily Journal Of Your Weight Loss Progress

Day Fifty Seven

Daily Journal Of Your Weight Loss Progress

Day Fifty Eight

DAILY JOURNAL OF YOUR WEIGHT LOSS PROGRESS

DAY FIFTY NINE

9251659R0

Made in the USA
Lexington, KY
14 April 2011